Chapter 1: My story, so far

CW00404227

My story is not a great one. It is not one of heroics and conquering with a fairy-tale ending. My story is one of identity, triumphs, though they may be small, fear and overcoming.

Hi, my name is Ella. I was born in 1999 with a condition called Microphthalmia (*microp thal mia*) and raised in the east of England with my mother and father, Diana and Nigel, and at least two cats at a time, we love our furry friends! I am sure my mother will agree that my birth was a traumatic one. While my mother was in labour I got stuck and while they began to prep for a c section I was born with the aid of forceps after over a day of labour. Rather than kicking and screaming I was limp and silent. The doctors believed that due to me getting stuck and their efforts to help me that my right arm was damaged to the point I would never be able to use it; my face was bruised and swelling because of the forceps going over the front and back of my head rather than the sides which left me with a permanent dent in my hairline that I can see and feel even now, and needing help to breathe for the first few minutes of my life and antibiotics at only minutes old. Under these circumstances I was taken away to the NICU right away to give me the medical care I would need and my parents didn't see me for the first couple of hours of my life. When they finally got the news that their little girl was okay and they could see me for the first time they were warned in hush tones beforehand.

"I am really sorry Mr and Mrs Bruce, I must tell you something before you see your daughter. I am sorry but she has a large birthmark on her hand"

My parents, who had just had to deal with the stress of a traumatic birth and seeing their seconds old daughter being carted away from them really... didn't care! Oh well, it's just a birthmark was the unanimous thoughts of my parents who were just so pleased that I was alive, unharmed and just a bit battered and bruised, and for my mother that those hours of tireless labour were finally over. When all of the chaos was over they were able to take me home and get on with normal life with a new born. That normality lasted all of a couple of days. When the bruising and swelling on my face started to go down my father began to notice that something wasn't quite right with one of my eyes. He saw that I wasn't opening my right eye the same as my left and that it looked a bit smaller or a different shape. When the health visitor came to see me for the first time, she agreed, something wasn't right. After going to our local GP, hospitals and health visitors, at five weeks old I was diagnosed with Microphthalmia. There was no hushed tones, no warning before the delivering blow, no final moment before the trajectory of my life, and theirs, would be changed just as it had begun. All I can think for my parents is that it must have been like the air being sucked from their lungs.

"As you know, Ella is blind in her right eye." And that was it.

From that moment we were put on a different path that we still strut down today!

Admittedly it wasn't plain sailing from there, we had lots to learn and many obstacles to pass. I was straight away referred to Moorefield's eye hospital in London where I would stay on their records until the age of 18 when I agreed to a partial discharge (meaning if I want or need to go back for any reason I can just call them and book an appointment without having to get referred to them again) so long as I had an optician keep a check on the health of both my eyes every year. Within the first few appointments at Moorfield's they confirmed that I also have Persistent Hyperplastic Primary Vitreous (PHPV), sometimes known as Persistent Fetal Vasculature (PFV). In very simple terms, when a baby is in the womb there is a liquid that covers and protects the front and back of the eye. This liquid is very similar to that which causes a cataract. In the weeks or days before birth and sometimes after birth, the liquid clears and goes away leaving normal sight for the baby. People with PHPV never have the liquid clear and turns in to a cataract which over the years will solidify. Thankfully after much testing they were able to confirm that my vision in my left eye was nearly perfect!

In 1999 there wasn't much in the way of resources available to the public about children born with microphthalmia or other ophthalmic conditions, that which my parents could find would be distressing medical accounts of worst-case scenarios. Today we are so lucky to have the ability to access the wide range of resources on any subject but unfortunately this has only been the case for the last ten years or so. All of these amazing charities, support pages and information sites were not available to my parents when I was born, they were faced with the very real possibility that I may never be able to function enough to have any independence, that I may never talk, that I may be extremely developmentally delayed, all of these 'possibilities', unanswered questions and lack of support must have felt like they were at sea without a life vest. In amongst all of this uncertainty the only 'support' my parents were given was a poem by Emily P Kingsley from 1987 entitled 'Welcome to Holland'. The poem talks about learning to accept that the birth of your child with a disability isn't what you had hoped or planned for, but it is still beautiful and with its charms. I am so glad that people nowadays, for any reason, have the ability to reach out for support in many different formats. I know for myself that being able to watch a video by someone who has the same medical condition as me, someone who understands what is happening to me and in my life, someone who may be a few years down the line or has experienced what I am going through now, that camaraderie and visibility continues to be such a comfort to me.

The next decade and a half of my life was pretty much the same series of events just in different orders at different times and in different ways. I remained in mainstream schools for all of my education and followed the natural progression of schooling. From the very start my family fought for me to be treated like any other student, not to be treated differently or given special accommodations because of my eye. We will cover the remainder of my school experience in later chapters.

Which brings us to today. I guess I should introduce myself again!

Hi, I'm Ella, my friends and colleagues call me El. In 2022 I am 23, I live with my partner and our adorable kitten Willow in a house we bought three days before my 23rd birthday. I currently work full time in the renewable and sustainable energy industry. I drive a non-adapted car which I passed my test for nine months exactly after my 17th birthday. In 2020 I graduated with a Bachelors of Arts with Honours in Philosophy from Anglia Ruskin University in Cambridge where I had lived for three years independently while studying. In September of 2021 I completed my Masters degree in History and in July of 2022 I finally got to have my graduation ceremony which Covid had to cruelly robbed me of before.

In 2018 I started uploading videos to YouTube about being a disabled student and my conditions. I continue to make videos about the things I find important and that make me happy. I like to consider myself an author and hopefully soon I will get the opportunity to impart the wisdom and knowledge I have gained on to the next generation and their families.

I feel that I must make a point before going any further.

Every person's experience is going to be different. Every family's experience is going to be different. As with all medical conditions it 100% varies from person to person and no two people will have the same symptoms, attributes and experiences even though they have the same medical conditions. Keeping this in mind, when reading this book please understand that this is my experience of my condition and may not mimic the experiences of your child. Take the advice and guidance you need and leave what you don't. I will also add that although I proudly call myself disabled, this is not because of my eye. Up until I was 14 I never considered myself disabled, my life was in no way effected by my health. When I was 14 I began developing symptoms of a genetic condition we didn't know I had and didn't find out about until I was 19. Later on we found that my mother's side of the family also have this condition, though milder than myself. It is our belief that my father's genetics acted as a catalyst to my mother's, causing my disability and it's subsequent symptoms. We were not and could not have been aware of this until over 20 years after my birth.

I hope my story helps you in the beginning chapters of your own.

Chapter 2: Getting (over) the news

Being told that there is something happening to your child that you have no power over is scary, confronting and confusing for anyone. The best piece of advice I can give you when faced with this situation is as follows;

GET OVER IT!

Don't ignore it, don't pretend it never happened, don't bury your head in the sand and wait for it to go away because it won't. Grab it by the horns, let yourself feel that fear and find away to get over it. Get over the fear, get over this hurdle of unknown, get over it and get on with life.

Of course, you can feel all of these emotions, you are human and you are 100% allowed to feel completely overwhelmed, but you need to feel it and move on. Each day you will feel it, you may feel like you are out of your depth and that you are doing the wrong thing, but each day you will find it a bit easier and each day you will know that you are doing the best you can. Maybe some days you will feel worse than the day before and maybe you will feel like its not any easier but it will never feel like its not 1000% worth it for your child.

I won't tell you that it will be okay and that you will come out of this being the best version of yourself and you will know all the right answers and all the right things to say and do. There will be work to do. You won't just be a parent. You will be a nurse, a medical receptionist, a driver to and from appointments, you'll be the person to hold their hand for blood test, you'll be a researcher, an advocate, someone to fight their corner and so much more.

When it comes to telling friends and family the news that you received you do not need to make it into anything more than something dropped into conversation. On the other hand, you do not need to hide it. If you start out by making it something that needs to be announced, something whispered and kept hush hush, a dirty word or something you become defensive about, your child will notice this and reflect your actions in their life. In the same way that they will start to feel like a part of them should be hidden away from society and be kept a secret, if you feel like you owe everyone in your life or that you meet an explanation and that you have to tell them right away your child will feel the same way about themselves. There may be people in yours and your child's life that you feel need to know about their condition, these maybe their immediate family or your closest friends and sometimes it does feel like if you can tell people that may be able to help you then it isn't as much of a weight on your shoulders.

No one at all is owed an explanation, no one deserves to know every detail about your child at all, know matter what their medical status is. Strangers, friends, family, anyone who is in your life or not. No one at all is owed any detail and you do not have to 'explain' your reasons for not telling them and they absolutely should respect your decision. If they start guessing, they do not respect you.

Keeping this in mind, there are two groups of people that I do believe should be told some level of detail, but that level is completely up to you and only you and eventually your child can decide what details they are given. This is the child's education system and the child's guardian's work. I will explain. If your child goes to mainstream school or a specialist school, it is always best to sit down with them before or as soon as possible with the school and your child and tell them three things:

1.
   What your child's condition/s are.
2.
   What this means for your child. Tell them your specific experience, don't give them the opportunity to google.
3.
   Tell them what your expectations are of them when it comes to how they treat and educate your child.

This way you know that if something happens when they are at school the relevant people understand the situation and how they can help. Make sure your child is present for this conversation, that way the people at the school can see how you and your child interact with each other. Be as honest as you can and remember to write everything down for them and that they add it to your child's file! That way, if staff leave and change and as your child goes through to different classes everyone will be able to access it. Remember, keep it updated. As you learn more about your child's condition and how it effects them, if they take medication, if they have issues with different situations. Let them know that you will need to take your child out of school for doctors appointments and that it cannot be helped, that you do not have choices of dates and times and that you will provide them with copies (do not give them the original letters, keep these safe in a file) as and when they come in. Give them a gentle reminder the week of/ week before the appointment.

When it comes to informing the child's guardian's work/ employment, I simply mean, have a brief conversation with a manager or supervisor, someone who approves your time off, let them know 'Hey, I will have to have time off to take my child to medical appointments as they have this condition. Sometimes my child may be unwell and I will have to be home with them, sometimes I may be able to work from home at these times and sometimes I won't because I will need to look after them all of the time. I will give you as much notice as possible for these appointments. I will send an email to you and HR reiterating this conversation so we are all informed as much as possible' by doing this they will hopefully understand that this time off is unavoidable and that the support you require from them is variable. By sending an email to both the person you talked to and your companies HR team, everyone is kept on the same page and there is less of a chance of miscommunication.

There is going to be people who feel like they deserve to give their opinion on your child and their condition. There is going to be people who think that it is comforting to you for them to tell you that their second cousins, dogs, aunt had a child that had a 'similar condition' and then go on to tell you all these horror stories. They don't matter. Their experiences do not matter to you. If they are not living it at that moment, if their intension is not to provide you with solidarity and comfort, they do not matter. Even if they are living it now and they are truly trying to comfort you and provide you with support, you still do not have to listen to them. You do not NEED anyone to tell you their experiences to help you with what is to come. Though there is strength and solidarity in sharing your experiences and trails with someone who can actually understand what it is you are dealing with. It is important to remember that everyone has different ways of handling and expressing their emotions.

If someone seems like they are 'handling' things better than you or is more emotional about their situation than you, it does not mean you are doing anything wrong or you don't care enough.

It is okay to feel your natural emotions because they are just that, natural, coming from nature. It is that same nature that makes your bond with your child so strong. It is also the same nature that caused your child to be born with this condition.

Reflect on that.

Chapter 3: Why me?

Sometimes this question is asked by the child themselves and sometimes its asked by the parent for themselves. 'why did this happen to me? Why my life?' or for their child 'what happened for it to happen to them? Why did this happen to them?'

In complete honesty, it doesn't matter how or why it happened because it has and no matter how much you wish it had happened to anyone else it won't change that.

It is difficult for parents who have found out at birth or after birth of their child who has a medical condition to not feel a sense of resentment towards their child. Of course, this is never something that is intentional, no parent wants to resent their child. There may come a point in your child's life where they resent you and blame you for their condition. The same way you don't mean it, they don't mean it either. It is not an easy road to go down, having to be so aware of your health, sometimes being in pain or frustrated because of your condition and it can be even worse if your condition is visible, sometimes you need something or someone to blame. Eventually they will be able to understand that it is your fault, it isn't their fault, it isn't anyone's fault.

Although it may be your personal prerogative to do so and it may be your own belief but try to avoid blaming or attributing your child's condition to a higher being. It has been well documented that children with medical conditions who are brought up in religious settings end up displaying religious trauma and a deep feeling of shame. If you wish to learn more about this, I suggest reading 'The Cultural and Religious Production of Disability Shame and the Saving Power of Heretical Bodies' by Michelle Mary Lelwica published in the Review of Disability Studies in 2019. Finding something that brings you comfort is okay, it is something that everyone searches for in times of stress and discomfort. It is important to remember that your comfort or coping mechanisms may be different to your child's as your experiences will be different.

When your child inevitably asks you the question 'why did this happen to me?' the best answer is always the honest one. If you have to tell your child that you don't know, then tell them you don't know. If you know what caused it be it genetics or environmental then tell them that. No matter what the answer is, tell them the truth. Children naturally ask why, it is likely that other children they interact with are asking why they are 'like this' and when they don't have the answers to give it can become overwhelming and start them asking these questions about themselves. It seems something so insignificant but communicating openly and honestly about your child's condition to them and with them from the beginning of their life will help to create the feeling of normalisation and trust.

With myself, my parents never called my right eye (the eye I am blind in) my poorly eye or my special eye, it has always been my small eye or blind eye because it is obviously smaller than my left eye.

Something that I always took comfort in is knowing that we are all different, no two people look the same, even twins have their differences. Humanity loves unique assurances, if you saw the same beautiful sunset every night you would eventually get tired of it and start to ignore its beauty. If you have ever looked at photos where they have mirrored one side of someone's face so they are completely symmetrical or a face that has been generated to be the perfect ratios, they are rather forgettable or unnerving. Our 'imperfections' is what makes us interesting and attractive. Nature is always creating unique events and objects, it is this which we find interesting and make us want to know what they are or how they came to be. We are always our own worst critic and we will never get to see ourselves through someone else's mind and eyes. That being said, it doesn't mean that people will always be able to appreciate our differences.

If faced with the question 'why did this happen to me? Why was I born blind and have a genetic condition that has made me disabled?', now at the age of 23, my answer is this:

If it wasn't me and my family, it would have been someone else. If it wasn't my life that was affected in this way, it would have been another baby born the same as me. It happened to me because I can handle it, my family could handle the situation we were placed in. I don't know 100% why I was born blind, it isn't genetic, we can speculate that it was environmental but at this point in my life I don't need to spend the time and energy answering that question because it wont change anything. Yes there have been times in my life where I have thought life would have been easier if I hadn't been born this way and there have been times when I was younger that I wished this was someone else's life. Eventually I have found myself coming to terms with my reality and learning that the foundations of my life are not going to change but the elements I choose to include in my life will.

My journey to this point has not been linear and I know that there may be points in the future where I may not feel the same way that I do now. I strongly believe that a pivotal point in my acceptance of myself and my reality was meeting people who had the same condition as me and looked like me. This helped me understand that I (and my family) are not alone and other people will have been thinking and feeling the same way that I did. I would strongly encourage trying to find other people who have the same condition as your child so that they can talk to other children who will be able to understand them. A great way to do this is to look for charities for specific conditions, go online or social media and try to find these charities and groups.

They will often have annual meetups or virtual events more frequently which will allow your children to socialise and get to know people like them as well as allowing you as the family to get to know other families that will have similar experiences to you.

Chapter 4: Getting on with getting on

No one, no book, no doctor, no friend, no family member, no random person who you definitely didn't ask their input, can tell you what is the best way to parent your child.

I cannot tell you what is going to happen in your child's life or what you should be doing to parent them in the best way possible. With most things it is trial and error to find what works for you and your child. However, I can give suggestions for how you can approach situations that will most likely arise for you with your child. These are my tips for as I like to say, getting on with getting on. This to me means powering through the things you don't necessarily want to deal with but have to deal with, normally with a forced smile.

1, When it comes doctors appointments, either try to find someone who isn't the child's immediate family to go with you or record the conversation and play it back to this person/people. This is so someone who isn't extremely emotionally invested (in the nicest way possible) can listen to what the doctor or medical professional has to say and can process that information in a logical way. It can be extremely emotional to hear news about your child that can sometimes lead to more questions than answers. We all have that person in our lives who is extremely organised, can handle high pressure situations, the kind of person we want to be with when an emergency happens. For me, that is my mum. Even now, at the age of 23, I prefer having my mother with me when I go to appointments because she is able to take in the information, ask the right questions and can then give me the information I need in a way I understand. Having someone like that with you at appointments, especially the first appointments when you are more likely to be given important information about your child's diagnosis and timeline of their condition/s, can be calming and very supportive.

2, If someone tells you your child can't do something, try! When I was born they didn't know if I would be able to walk properly because they thought my balance was going to be extremely poor. They didn't know if I would be able to write because they didn't think I would know where the paper was and not know where I was putting the pen. All of these and so many more limitations my teachers put on me could have stopped me from trying. If I hadn't tried, I never would have known all the amazing things I could do. Of course some of the ways I learnt how to do things were different to other children, but if we are all aiming for the same destination, does it matter how we get there?

3, Find something that they enjoy and are "good at". It can be literally anything, if possible an activity they can do alone or don't have to rely on anyone else for. This will give them something to focus on when other elements of their life feel hard. it can provide a sense of independence and over coming. It can also provide the notion of "well at least I have…"

4, Use the scientific/ biologically correct language when refereeing to your child and their condition. By giving them the correct language this will give them the ability to talk to adults in a clear and informative manner and aid in the case of a medical or emergency situation. This will also aid in normalising their condition not only for you and your child but for those you talk to frequently. It will also mean that as they grow up they will be able to understand more of their medical care and can potentially alleviate medical anxiety as they feel more informed and in control of their situation.

5, Have weekly check ins. A check in is a time where you come together with your child and ask them how they are. Not only medically but emotionally and mentally. These check ins don't have to be an intervention, it can be sat having breakfast or in the car on the way to school, so long as it is a place where they feel safe and they can express themselves without fear of being judged. A great way to get them to open up is to take part in the check ins too. They will be able to see that you are being open and honest and they will think that it is just a part of normal life. The idea of this is to create a foundation and a routine of talking about how they feel both physically and emotionally. It is known that people who fall into a minority category experience mental health issues at a higher degree or more frequently than those who do not.

6, always have something to be getting on with. Hobbies and clubs are so important to all children but they really become a great distraction tool for children who maybe faced with personal struggles. Having something that I was able to put myself into, something that meant I wasn't going only between home and school, meant that I was able to forget about the other elements of my life for a moment and focus completely on what I was doing right then. From my own experience, having something that made me leave the house and go somewhere and participate with other people, as well as having a hobby that I could do at home, by myself, whenever I wanted for how long I wanted, meant that at any time if I needed that escape I could have it. It also meant that on days when I really didn't want to be with other kids but I also didn't want to have to spend all day with my parents I had something I could enjoy independently. This mix of activities proved exceptionally helpful to me and is something I will be implementing for my own children regardless. For children who spend most of their days feeling like they aren't entirely excepted, don't have much independence or maybe haven't ever felt part of a friend group or a team, having something that is yours, away from parents and teachers, will be not only a massive self-esteem boost, but also a great teaching moment for independence, tolerance and acceptance.

My biggest piece of advise is this; trust yourself. You know that all you want is the very best for your child. There will be days where you feel under equipped but with everything, it will pass.

Chapter 5: What now?

I can't say what is to come now. I can't say that one day the answers that you need or want will appear in front of you. Even now, over 20 years later we still don't know why I was born the way I was. We don't know if we will ever know. We have made our peace with that. But something we do know is that if we do not look for the answers, if we do not do what we can and search for them, we will never find them. My family and I still take part in studies, we give blood, answer questionnaires, anything we can to help. Even if we don't get answers but someone else does, its worth it.

There are still aspects of my life that are, not difficult, are different because of my eye. Other people probably don't even notice because I do them as second nature. It is always easier to be born different, than to develop it over time. I am so glad that I never had sight in my right eye. I am so glad that I have never known life other than this. When I learnt to walk, I learnt with only vision in one eye. When I learnt to ride a bike, I learnt with only vision in one eye. When I learnt to drive, I learnt with only vision in one eye. I didn't have to relearn anything. I didn't have to grieve loosing something, because I didn't have it in the first place. Some people pity me for that. Because I never knew anything different. I have never had the opportunity to see the world the same as everyone else. I never had the opportunity to be 'normal'. I also never had the opportunity to loose my sight. My parents and I didn't have the option to worry about what was going to happen, because it already happened before I was born. I didn't have to change my life, because this is the life I started with. There is nothing that I have to do differently from how I have always lived. I am grateful for that.

Everything I have said throughout this book is just my own thoughts, feels and experiences. Because blindness is such a varied condition there is no set plan to follow that leads to the perfect out come. Every child and every family will face their own set of challenges, you have to learn to navigate your own. I just hope that this has been of some help. You have access to a wide range of resources. There are other people like me out there who talk about their experience and help share tips for ways you can support your child through this aspect of their life.

Even now in to my 20's I still face things in my life that would be easier if I wasn't born like this. Sometimes I wish I didn't have to deal with the appointments, the doctors visits, the comments. But I remind myself. It's not everyday. It's not every comment. It's not every person. I get to be who I am, I get to share my life and my story and bring comfort to those who have entered the darkest moments of their life. I get to show people that it will be okay, and I will take that and the annoying parts every day.

I also remind myself that I do not owe anyone advocacy. Just because I was born this way and it was decided for me, it doesn't also mean that advocacy was decided for me. I choose to do this because I can and I want to. You do not owe anyone visibility or advocacy and neither does your child. That is for you and them to decide.

I wish I could tell you that it will be easy, that your life won't be affected by this and that your child we thrive the same as any other child. But I can't. I can't tell you that, especially in the beginning, it won't be hard, that it won't be heart breaking or hopeless. What I can tell you is that your life will be affected in amazing ways, as well as some harder ones. That nothing great is ever easy. That your child will thrive in their own way and it will be such a gift to watch that.

 I can tell you, with everything I know, that it will always be worth it.

Printed in Great Britain
by Amazon

41952835R00020